CU01083805

The Newly Complete Galveston Diet Cookbook for Starter's 2023

The Healthy Delicious Guide to Lose Weight Quickly, Improve Blood Sugar Control And Manage Inflammation.

Khloe Cocker

TABLE OF CONTENTS

INTRODUCTION

The Galveston Diet is based on the idea that a diet high in whole, unprocessed plant foods can improve overall health and help prevent chronic diseases such as heart disease, diabetes, and cancer. The diet is rich in fruits, vegetables, whole grains, and legumes, and is low in saturated fats and added sugars.

In this book, you will find a variety of recipes that are inspired by the flavors and ingredients of Galveston but have been adapted to fit the principles of the Galveston Diet. From breakfast dishes like "Galveston Island Tofu Scramble" and "Sweet Potato Hash with Black Beans and Avocado," to lunch and dinner options like "Vegetable Jambalaya" and "Gulf Coast Grilled

Portobello Mushrooms," there is something for every taste and preference.

In addition to recipes, the book will also include tips on how to stock a plant-based pantry, how to make substitutions in recipes, and how to make the most of your leftovers. Each recipe includes a nutritional breakdown and a list of ingredients, as well as step-by-step instructions for easy preparation.

The Galveston Diet is not just about weight loss, it's about improving your overall health and well-being. The recipes in this book are designed to make it easy for you to incorporate the principles of the Galveston Diet into your everyday life. Whether you are looking to improve your health, lose weight, or simply want to eat delicious and nutritious meals, this book has something for you. So let's get started on our journey to healthy and delicious eating with Galveston Diet Recipes!

In addition to the delicious and healthy recipes, this book also includes information on the history and culture of Galveston, and how it has influenced the local cuisine. Galveston, located on the Gulf of Mexico, has a rich history as a port city and a melting pot of cultures, which has led to a diverse and flavorful cuisine. The local seafood, such as shrimp, crab, and oysters, as well as the abundance of fresh fruits and vegetables grown in the area, have played a major role in shaping the local cuisine.

One of the key features of the Galveston Diet is its emphasis on whole, unprocessed foods. This means that the recipes in this book use minimally processed ingredients and rely on fresh, natural flavors to create delicious and satisfying meals. We also provide alternative suggestions for those who are gluten-free, nut-free, and soy-free.

Another important aspect of the Galveston Diet is its emphasis on eating in moderation. Many of the recipes in this book are designed to be lower in calories, while still providing the nutrients your body needs. This means you can enjoy larger portions of your favorite meals without feeling guilty.

In addition to the recipes, the book also includes a section on tips and tricks for making the most of your leftovers, meal planning, and pantry essentials. This will help you save time and money, and reduce food waste.

Overall, this book is a great resource for anyone looking to improve their health and well-being through a plant-based diet. By incorporating the principles of the Galveston Diet into your daily life, you will be able to enjoy delicious and nutritious meals that are inspired by the flavors and ingredients of Galveston. So, let's dive into the world of Galveston Diet Recipes and start enjoying the delicious and healthy way of life today!

CHAPTER ONE

The key Components of the Galveston Diet, including its focus on Anti-inflammatory foods and Intermittent fasting

One of the key components of the Galveston Diet is its emphasis on anti-inflammatory foods. Inflammation is a natural response of the body to injury or infection, but chronic inflammation has been linked to some health conditions, including heart disease, diabetes, and cancer. The Galveston Diet promotes the consumption of foods that are known to have anti-inflammatory properties, such as fruits, vegetables, whole grains, and legumes. These foods are rich in antioxidants, phytochemicals, and other nutrients that can help to reduce inflammation and promote overall health.

Another key component of the Galveston Diet is its emphasis on intermittent fasting. Intermittent fasting is a method of eating in which you alternate between periods of eating and periods of fasting. The Galveston Diet suggests that by limiting the time during which you eat, you can improve your body's ability to burn fat and improve overall health. In addition, intermittent fasting has been shown to have several health benefits, such as reducing inflammation, improving insulin sensitivity, and reducing the risk of chronic diseases.

The Galveston Diet also emphasizes the importance of avoiding processed foods, added sugars, and unhealthy fats. These foods can be high in calories, low in nutrients, and can contribute to inflammation and chronic diseases. Instead, the diet encourages the consumption of whole foods that are nutrient-dense and provide the body with the vitamins, minerals, and nutrients it needs for optimal health.

In summary, the Galveston Diet is a dietary plan that focuses on anti-inflammatory foods, intermittent fasting, and the consumption of whole, nutrient-dense foods. By following this diet, individuals can improve their overall health and reduce their risk of chronic diseases. It is important to note, however, that before starting any new dietary plan, it is always best to consult with a healthcare professional to ensure it is safe and appropriate for you.

Another important aspect of the Galveston Diet is its emphasis on portion control. The diet encourages individuals to eat until they are satisfied, rather than until they are full. Overeating and weight gain can be avoided in this way. Additionally, the diet suggests that individuals should eat at regular intervals throughout the day, rather than skipping meals or eating large meals infrequently. This can help to regulate blood sugar levels and reduce feelings of hunger.

The Galveston Diet also includes many specific food recommendations. For example, it suggests that individuals consume at least 8-10 servings of fruits and vegetables each day. These foods are rich in nutrients and antioxidants and can help to reduce inflammation and promote overall health. In addition, the diet recommends that individuals consume at least 3 servings of whole grains each day, such as quinoa, brown rice, and whole wheat. Whole grains are high in fiber and provide a variety of important nutrients, such as B vitamins, iron, and zinc.

One of the most important aspects of the Galveston Diet is its focus on plant-based foods. The diet encourages individuals to consume a wide variety of plant-based foods, such as fruits, vegetables, whole grains, legumes, and nuts. These foods are low in saturated fat and cholesterol and are high in fiber and nutrients. By consuming a diet that is rich in plant-based foods, individuals can reduce their risk of chronic diseases, such as heart disease and cancer, and improve their overall health.

The Galveston Diet is a dietary plan that focuses on anti-inflammatory foods, intermittent fasting, and the consumption of whole, nutrient-dense foods. It emphasizes the importance of portion control and regular meals, the consumption of fruits, vegetables, whole grains, and legumes, and the reduction of processed foods, added sugars, and unhealthy fats. By following this diet, individuals can improve their overall health, reduce their risk of chronic diseases and lose weight if necessary. However, as with any dietary change, it is important to speak with a healthcare professional to ensure it is safe and appropriate for you.

How to Set your Optimum Macronutrient and Calorie Objectives

Determining your ideal calorie and macronutrient goals is an important step in achieving a healthy and sustainable diet. There are several factors to consider when setting these goals, including your age, gender, weight, activity level, and overall health.

First, it's important to understand the difference between calories and macronutrients. Calories are a unit of measure for energy, while macronutrients are the three main nutrients that provide energy: carbohydrates, proteins, and fats. Each macronutrient has a specific calorie value per gram: carbohydrates and proteins contain 4 calories per gram, while fats contain 9 calories per gram.

To determine your ideal calorie goal, you can use a calorie calculator or consult with a registered dietitian. Generally, the average adult needs between 1,200 and 2,500 calories per day, depending on their activity level and overall health. Factors such as weight loss or gain, pregnancy, or certain medical conditions may require a different calorie goal.

Next, you should determine your macronutrient goals. The ideal macronutrient ratio will vary depending on your personal goals and dietary preferences. For example, a high-carbohydrate diet is often recommended for athletes who need a lot of energy for endurance training, while a high-protein diet may be recommended for those looking to build muscle mass. A diet that is high in fats may be recommended for those looking to lose weight or improve brain function.

A general recommendation is to aim for a diet that is 45-65% carbohydrates, 10-35%

protein, and 20-35% fat. However, it's important to note that these recommendations are not one-size-fits-all and should be adjusted based on your individual needs and goals.

It's important to remember that calorie and macronutrient goals are not set in stone and may need to be adjusted as your body changes over time. Regularly monitoring your progress and consulting with a registered dietitian or healthcare professional can help ensure that your goals are appropriate and realistic.

It's also important to keep in mind that calorie restriction for weight loss is not always the best approach, as it can lead to nutrient deficiencies, muscle loss, and a slower metabolism. Instead, it is advisable to focus on nutrient-dense foods and a balanced diet, along with the regular physical activity.

Determining your ideal calorie and macronutrient goals is an important step in achieving a healthy and sustainable diet. It involves considering your age, gender, weight, activity level, and overall health. A calorie calculator or a consultation with a registered dietitian can help you determine your ideal calorie goal. macronutrient goals should be based on your personal goals and dietary preferences. Remember that calorie and macronutrient goals are not set in stone and may need to be adjusted as your body changes over time. Regularly monitoring your progress and consulting with a healthcare professional can help ensure that your goals are appropriate and realistic.

Once you have determined your ideal calorie and macronutrient goals, it's important to track your intake to ensure that you are meeting them. There are several ways to do this, including using a food diary, a mobile app, or an online tool. These tools can help you track the number of calories and macronutrients you are consuming each day and make adjustments as needed.

It's also important to consider the quality of the calories and macronutrients you are consuming. There are variations among calories and macronutrients. For example, a diet high in processed foods and added sugars may provide a lot of calories, but it may also be lacking in essential nutrients. On the other hand, a diet rich in whole foods such as fruits, vegetables, lean protein, and healthy fats may provide fewer calories but will be more nutrient-dense.

Additionally, it's important to keep in mind that your body's needs may change depending on the day. For example, if you have a day of heavy physical activity, you may need to consume more calories and carbohydrates to fuel your body. On the other hand, if you have a more sedentary day, you may need to consume fewer calories to avoid overeating.

Finally, it's also important to remember that weight loss and weight gain are not always the only goals for setting calorie and macronutrient goals. Other factors such as overall health, energy levels, and disease management should also be considered. For example, for people with type 2 diabetes, a diet high in healthy fats and low in carbohydrates may be more beneficial in managing blood sugar levels than a low-fat diet.

Intermittent Fasting Pros & Cons

Intermittent fasting (IF) is a pattern of eating where a person alternates between periods of eating and fasting. It is not a diet in the traditional sense, as it does not specify which foods to eat or avoid, but rather when to eat. The most popular forms of IF include the 16/8 method, where a person fasts for 16 hours and eats during an 8-hour window, and the 5:2 diet, where a person eats normally for 5 days and restricts calories to 500-600 for the other 2 non-consecutive days.

IF has been gaining popularity in recent years for its potential health benefits. One of the main benefits is weight loss, as it can lead to a reduction in calorie intake and an increase in fat burning. Studies have also shown that IF can improve insulin sensitivity, lower inflammation, and improve heart health markers. Additionally, it may have benefits for cognitive function, such as increasing focus and concentration, and may even have anti-aging effects.

It's important to note that intermittent fasting may not be suitable for everyone, especially for women with a history of disordered eating, pregnant or breastfeeding women, people with a history of eating disorders, people with diabetes, and people who have had or have a history of gastrointestinal issues.

It's also important to be mindful of your nutrient intake during the eating periods. While intermittent fasting can lead to weight loss, it's not an excuse to eat unhealthy foods during the eating periods. It's important to continue to eat a balanced diet that is rich in fruits, vegetables, whole grains, lean proteins, and healthy fats.

Intermittent fasting is a pattern of eating that can have potential health benefits but it's not suitable for everyone. It's important to speak with a healthcare professional before starting any new eating pattern and to be mindful of nutrient intake during the eating periods. It's also important to remember that intermittent fasting is not a magic solution for weight loss, it's important to maintain a healthy lifestyle with a balanced diet, regular physical activity, and sufficient sleep.

Anti-Inflammatory Nutrition Approach

Anti-inflammatory nutrition is a dietary approach that focuses on consuming foods that have been shown to have anti-inflammatory properties.

Although inflammation is a typical immunological response to injury or infection, persistent inflammation has been linked to the emergence of some illnesses, including cancer, heart disease, and autoimmune disorders.

By eating a diet full of anti-inflammatory foods, one of the main objectives of anti-inflammatory nutrition is to lower the body's overall levels of inflammation. These foods consist of:

Fruits And Vegetables: It has been shown that the antioxidants, vitamins, and minerals included in fruits and vegetables have anti-inflammatory qualities. While leafy greens, broccoli, and cauliflower are rich in anti-inflammatory substances, berries, cherries, and tomatoes are especially strong in antioxidants.

Fish like salmon and tuna, as well as flaxseeds, chia seeds, and walnuts, are good sources of omega-3 fatty acids. It has been shown that these fatty acids help to lessen bodily inflammation.

Whole grains: Whole grains are high in fiber and anti-inflammatory chemicals. Examples of such grains are quinoa, barley, and oats. There is evidence that they lower the chance of developing heart disease and other chronic illnesses.

Herbs and spices: Turmeric, ginger, and rosemary are among the herbs and spices that are high in anti-inflammatory components. They have been used for many years in conventional treatment to lessen inflammation and advance general wellness.

Nuts and seeds: Nuts and seeds, such as almonds, walnuts, and pumpkin seeds, are a great source of healthful fats and anti-inflammatory substances. They are a wonderful meat substitute for vegetarians and vegans since they are a rich source of protein.

On the other hand, several nutrients and foods have been linked to a higher risk of inflammation. These consist of:

Foods that have been processed: It has been shown that eating foods that have been processed cause the body's inflammatory response to rising.

Refined carbs: Refined carbohydrates have been deprived of their essential nutrients and fiber, white bread, and pasta. They enter the circulation fast, causing an increase in blood sugar and inflammation.

Trans fats: It has been shown that trans fats, which are included in many processed foods, cause the body to become more inflammatory. These should be kept as far away as possible.

Alcohol: Drinking too much alcohol may cause organ inflammation, including in the liver.

High-sugar Foods: Chronic inflammation and the generation of pro-inflammatory chemicals are both connected to high-sugar diets.

Consuming foods with anti-inflammatory qualities, such as fruits and vegetables, omega-3 fatty acids, whole grains, spices, herbs, nuts, and seeds, is the main goal of anti-inflammatory nutrition, a dietary strategy. To manage inflammation in the body, it's also crucial to stay away from processed meals, refined carbs, trans fats, alcohol, and foods rich in sugar. It is crucial to remember that the secret to maximizing the benefits and maintaining general health is a well-balanced diet that contains a range of anti-inflammatory foods.

In conclusion, setting your ideal macronutrient and calorie objectives is a crucial step in developing a diet that is both wholesome and sustainable. It needs frequent monitoring and modifications and takes into account factors like your age, gender, weight, amount of exercise, and general health. Utilizing a food diary or mobile app to track your consumption will help you make sure that you are accomplishing your objectives. For general health, the quality of calories and macronutrients is also crucial. The ultimate objective of calories and macronutrients objectives should include managing diseases and general health as well as weight growth or reduction.

Creating wholesome, balanced meals that adhere to the Galveston Diet's rules may be done with the help of some meal-planning advice.

CHAPTER TWO:

Advice for Meal Preparation on the Galveston Diet

A healthy weight may be attained and maintained by a weight reduction regimen like the Galveston Diet, which emphasizes eating balanced, nutrient-rich meals. The diet is predicated on the notion that by eating a mix of lean proteins, complex carbs, and healthy fats, you may lower your chance of developing chronic illnesses and enhance your general health.

Meal preparation is a crucial part of the Galveston Diet. You can make sure you are getting a balance of nutrients and adhering to the diet's rules by taking the time to prepare your meals in advance. Here are some suggestions to assist you in preparing healthy, balanced meals that adhere to the **Galveston Diet's Rules:**

Plan your meals so that you may be sure to have all the ingredients on hand and avoid being tempted to eat unhealthy foods.

Include A Variety Of Nutrients: The Galveston Diet stresses the value of eating a variety of lean proteins, complex carbs, and healthy fats. Make sure each meal has a supply of complex carbs like quinoa or sweet potatoes, a source of lean protein like chicken or fish, and a source of healthy fat like avocado or almonds.

Variety of fruits and vegetables should be included: Following the Galveston Diet, consuming since they are abundant in vitamins, minerals, and antioxidants, a range of fruits and vegetables. To ensure that you are receiving a broad range of nutrients, try to incorporate a variety of fruits and vegetables in your meals.

Reduce Your Intake Of Processed Foods: These foods are often heavy in salt, saturated fat, and added sugars, which may lead to chronic illnesses. Instead, choose nutrient-rich whole meals that have not been processed.

Try out some new recipes to keep things fresh and avoid becoming tired with your meals. Look for meals that employ entire, unprocessed products and integrate a balance of nutrients.

You may prepare nutritious, well-balanced meals that adhere to the Galveston Diet's rules by using the advice in this article. To succeed on this diet, keep in mind that planning your meals and concentrating on nutrient-dense, whole foods are essential.

And be sure to speak with a licensed healthcare practitioner before making any significant dietary adjustments.

When planning your meals, it's crucial to keep portion sizes in mind since getting too much of any one vitamin may be bad for your health. The Galveston Diet advises measuring portions by the size of your hand. A portion of healthy fats should be approximately the size of your thumb, a serving of protein about the size of your palm, and a serving of carbs about the size of your fist.

Use Nutritious Cooking Techniques: Food preparation has a big influence on nutritional content. Consider employing healthy cooking techniques such as grilling, baking, steaming, or sautéing to improve the nutritional value of your meals. Avoid techniques that call for using a lot of oil or deep frying.

Eating consciously and paying attention to hunger and fullness signals are two things that the Galveston diet promotes. Being present when you eat, enjoying each mouthful, and paying attention to your body's cues for fullness are all examples of mindful eating. This is a fantastic approach to curbing your appetite and becoming more in touch with your body's natural cues of hunger and fullness.

Eat With Others: Eating with others not only promotes social interaction but may also assist you in maintaining a healthy diet. You are less likely to overeat or choose unhealthy foods when you dine with others.

Be Flexible: The Galveston Diet is flexible, so it's crucial to keep in mind that it's OK to sometimes indulge in a treat or skip a meal. The secret is to keep your diet balanced and consistent over time.

You will be able to prepare meals that are nutritious, and balanced, and adhere to the Galveston Diet rules by paying attention to these suggestions and adopting them into your daily routine. To succeed on this diet, keep in mind that planning your meals and concentrating on nutrient-dense, whole foods are essential. And be sure to speak with a licensed healthcare practitioner before making any significant dietary adjustments.

Recipes for breakfast, lunch, supper, and dessert, as well as suggestions for nutritious snacks.

The Galveston Diet is a low-carb, high-fat eating plan that emphasizes vegetables, lean protein, and healthy fats while restricting the use of grains, sweets, and processed foods. The diet's objectives are to encourage weight reduction, enhance general health, and lower the chance of developing chronic illnesses.

Here are some ideas for making nutritious, well-balanced meals that adhere to the Galveston Diet:

Emphasize Good Fats: The Galveston Diet places a lot of emphasis on healthy fats such as olive oil, avocado, almonds, and seeds. These fats give off energy and help fat-soluble vitamins to be absorbed. Use olive oil when cooking, add avocado to salads and sandwiches, and add nuts and seeds as a snack or topping to your food to include healthy fats.

Include Protein: The Galveston Diet places a strong emphasis on getting adequate protein. Meat, fish, eggs, and lentils are all excellent sources of protein. To feel full and satisfied between meals, try to incorporate a protein-rich food.

Consume A Lot Of Veggies; they are a fantastic option for the Galveston Diet since they are low in carbohydrates and rich in fiber. Try to include a variety of vegetables, such as bell peppers, broccoli, cauliflower, and leafy greens, in your meals.

In advance: The Galveston Diet must be followed with meticulous planning and preparation of meals. Create sure you have all the supplies on hand and make your meals in advance. You may save time and maintain your diet by preparing your meals in advance.

Snacks are permitted on the Galveston Diet, but it's crucial to choose nutritious ones. Nuts, seeds, hard-boiled eggs, and veggies with dip are a few healthy options.

Here are some Galveston Diet-compliant dishes for breakfast, lunch, supper, and dessert:

Breakfast:

Egg and Avocado Breakfast bowl with mashed avocado, tomatoes, and a fried egg on top.

Cooked bacon and sautéed spinach are added to beaten eggs in a bacon and spinach omelet.

Lunch:

Grilled Chicken Salad: Place grilled chicken, avocado, and vinaigrette dressing on top of mixed greens.

Lettuce wraps with tuna salad: Combine canned tuna, mayonnaise, and sliced celery. Use lettuce cups to serve.

Dinner:

Salmon fillet that has been baked with roasted veggies on the side. The salmon fillet has been baked with a lemon and herb flavor.

Beef and Broccoli Stir-Fry: Marinate beef in garlic, ginger, and coconut aminos before stirring-frying it with broccoli and serving it over cauliflower rice.

Dessert:

Make chocolate coconut fat bombs by combining coconut oil, cocoa powder, and your preferred sweetener. Ballize the mixture, then freeze.

Berry Cheesecake: Combine cream cheese, vanilla essence, and your preferred sweetener. Spread the mixture over the crushed-nut crust, and then sprinkle the berries on top.

You may prepare nutritious, balanced meals that are in line with the Galveston Diet, encourage weight reduction, and improve general health by using these suggestions and recipes.

On the Galveston Diet, you may consume things like:

Meat: The Galveston Diet permits the consumption of all sorts of meat, including beef, hog, chicken, and fish. These meals are thought to have a low carbohydrate content while being rich in protein.

Vegetables: The Galveston Diet permits the use of vegetables such as leafy greens, broccoli, cauliflower, and peppers. These meals are rich in vitamins and minerals and have few carbs.

Dairy: On the Galveston Diet, dairy items like cheese, butter, and cream are permitted. These foods are regarded as having low carbohydrate content and being rich in fat and protein.

Nuts And Seeds: The Galveston Diet permits nuts and seeds such as almonds, pecans, and sunflower seeds. These foods are regarded as having low carbohydrate content and being rich in fat and protein.

Healthy Fats: The Galveston Diet permits the use of healthy fats including olive oil, avocado, and coconut oil. These meals are said to be low in carbs and a great source of energy.

The following foods are prohibited on the Galveston Diet:

Sugars and sweets: The Galveston Diet forbids the use of sugar, candy, and other sweets. These meals contain a lot of carbs and may raise blood sugar levels.

Grain: The Galveston Diet forbids the use of grains such as wheat, rice, and maize. These meals contain a lot of carbs and may raise blood sugar levels.

Legumes: The Galveston Diet forbids the consumption of legumes such as beans, lentils, and peas. These meals contain a lot of carbs and may raise blood sugar levels.

Fruits: According to the Galveston Diet, fruit is not permitted. Fruits contain a lot of carbs and may raise blood sugar levels.

Starchy Veggies: The Galveston Diet forbids the use of starchy vegetables including potatoes, sweet potatoes, and yams. These meals contain a lot of carbs and may raise blood sugar levels.

It's crucial to keep in mind that this diet may be restricted, that it can be challenging to follow for an extended time, that it may not be the ideal strategy for everyone, and that it's always a good idea to speak with a healthcare expert before beginning any diet program.

Other advantages of the Galveston diet for health

The Galveston Diet may help with blood sugar regulation, which is one of its main health advantages. To decrease blood sugar levels, a high-fat, low-carb diet reduces the quantity of glucose (sugar) in the blood. As it may enhance insulin sensitivity and lessen the need for medication, this can be very helpful for those with type 2 diabetes.

The capacity of the Galveston Diet to enhance cardiovascular health is another possible health advantage. The diet may help reduce cholesterol and triglyceride levels, which may minimize the risk of heart disease, by limiting the consumption of refined carbs and increasing the intake of good fats.

The Galveston Diet has also been shown to have a favorable effect on neurological health. The ketogenic components of the diet may enhance cognitive function and provide defense against neurological diseases like Parkinson's and Alzheimer's.

Certain kinds of cancer patients may potentially benefit from the Galveston diet. The ketogenic components of the diet may aid in limiting the development and division of cancer cells.

It's crucial to remember that not everyone should follow the Galveston Diet, especially if they have specific medical issues or dietary limitations. Any large dietary changes should always be discussed with a healthcare professional.

The Galveston Diet may help with weight reduction, but it also has additional advantages for your health, including better blood sugar regulation, cardiovascular and neurological health, and a potential influence on certain cancer types. However, it's always advisable to speak with a medical expert before making any significant dietary adjustments.

CHAPTER THREE

Shopping for Galveston Diet-friendly Foods

A low-carb, high-fat diet called the Galveston Diet is intended to encourage weight reduction and enhance general health. It's crucial to follow the diet to Choose the correct meals and stay away from those that are forbidden.

When purchasing foods that are appropriate for the Galveston Diet, seek whole, unadulterated foods such as meats, fish, eggs, veggies, and healthy fats. Some of the top stores to buy these foods are listed below:

Local Farmers' Markets: Farmers' markets provide a large range of in-season, fresh produce that is obtained locally. These foods often include no preservatives or additives and are frequently less priced than those bought at supermarkets.

Specialty meat and fish stores often have a larger assortment of premium, sustainably sourced meats, and seafood than supermarkets. Additionally, the meat and fish at these markets often come in a range of cuts and varieties, making it simple to locate what you want.

Foods that are organic, non-GMO, and gluten-free may be found in abundance at health food shops like Whole Foods. These shops often provide a wider variety of substitute sweeteners and flours that may be used in recipes instead of regular sugar and flour.

Online Grocery Buying: Online grocery shopping is getting more and more common these days. For those with restricted time or mobility, many online grocers provide a greater variety of items than conventional supermarkets.

Tips For Grocery Shopping:

A label check is a must if purchasing processed goods.

Avoid meals that have a lot of artificial chemicals and extra sugars.

To prevent impulsive purchases, make a list of the foods you need and stick to them.

Utilize special offers and specials to reduce your shopping expenditure.

Allowable Meals:

eggs, fish, and meat

Non-starchy veggies including bell peppers, broccoli, cauliflower, and leafy greens

Healthy fats include avocado, coconut, and olive oil, for instance.

seeds and nuts

dairy goods like heavy cream, butter, and cheese

Grains including oats, rice, and wheat are prohibited foods.

Sweeteners and sugars

in starchy foods like corn and potatoes

processed snacks and foods

Bananas, grapes, and pineapple are among the fruits that are rich in carbs.

You may effectively follow the Galveston Diet and accomplish your weight reduction and health objectives by adhering to these recommendations and choosing the correct things to eat.

Here are some additional considerations to make while looking for foods that are suitable for the Galveston Diet in addition to the advice and lists already provided:

In advance: Make a weekly food plan before you go grocery shopping. By doing this, you can ensure that you have all the required materials on hand and avoid making needless purchases.

Stock Up On Pantry Essentials: Some ingredients, like nuts, seeds, and olive oil, are wonderful to have on hand since they can be used in several dishes. Stock up on these things so that you always have access to them.

Embrace Experimentation: The Galveston Diet permits a broad range of meals, so don't be hesitant to explore new dishes and ingredients. This may help minimize boredom and keep your meals exciting.

Take Advantage Of Discounts: Meats, fruits, and vegetables that are about to expire are often discounted at stores. These meals may be consumed immediately or frozen.

Even though the Galveston Diet permits high-fat meals, it's still vital to pay attention to portion amounts. Even eating wholesome foods in excess might result in weight gain.

Beware Of Hidden Carbohydrates: Even typically healthful items like yogurt and salad dressings may include additional sugars or other substances that add carbs. Make sure an item is indeed suitable for the Galveston Diet by carefully reading the nutrition label and ingredient list.

You may easily traverse the grocery store and choose the healthiest meals for the Galveston Diet by keeping these suggestions in mind and being aware of the authorized and prohibited items. Keep in mind that the

Galveston Diet is a lifestyle change, therefore it's critical to maintain consistency and diversity in your meals to make them more pleasurable and sustainable.

Using the Galveston Diet's essential kitchen tools and methods are covered in Chapter 4.

A low-carb, high-fat diet called the Galveston Diet is intended to encourage weight reduction and enhance general health. It's crucial to have a solid grasp of the fundamental cooking equipment and methods to successfully follow this diet. This chapter will provide you with a general overview of the methods and equipment you'll need to successfully implement the Galveston Diet, as well as detailed instructions for preparing meals.

CHAPTER FOUR

Important Kitchenware

Cutting board: An important element of kitchenware is a cutting board. Having a sturdy, a sizable cutting board is essential for meal preparation.

Knives: The Galveston Diet requires you to prepare all of your meals using a decent set of knives. A serrated knife, a paring knife, and a chef's knife are necessary.

Measuring Cups And Spoons: Measuring cups and spoons are necessary for accurately measuring ingredients for your meals.

Mixing Bowls: Mixing bowls are essential for mixing ingredients and preparing food.

Pots and pans: Pots and pans are necessary for cooking your meals on the Galveston

Diet. It is important to have a variety of sizes and types of pots and pans to accommodate different cooking methods.

Skillet: A skillet is a great tool for cooking a variety of foods on the Galveston Diet.

Slow cooker: A slow cooker is a great tool for preparing meals on the Galveston Diet. It allows you to prepare meals in advance and have them ready when you get home.

Tongs: Tongs are useful for flipping food while cooking and serving food.

Whisk: A whisk is essential for mixing ingredients and preparing food.

Cooking Techniques

Baking: Baking is a great cooking technique for the Galveston Diet. It allows you to cook food without adding extra fats or oils.

Boiling: Boiling is a great cooking technique for the Galveston Diet. You can quickly and simply prepare meals using it.

Grilling: Grilling is a great cooking technique for the Galveston Diet. It allows you to cook food without adding extra fats or oils.

Roasting: Roasting is a great cooking technique for the Galveston Diet. It allows you to cook food without adding extra fats or oils.

Sautéing: Sautéing is a great cooking technique for the Galveston Diet. It allows you to quickly and easily make meals.

Stir-frying: Stir-frying is a great cooking technique for the Galveston Diet. It enables you to prepare meals fast and simply.

Making the Most of Leftovers

Use leftovers to make new meals:
Leftovers can be used to make new meals,
such as frittatas, omelets, soups, and salads.
Repurpose leftovers into new dishes:
Leftovers can be repurposed into new
dishes, such as sandwiches, pizzas, and
burritos.

Freeze leftovers for later: Leftovers can
be frozen for later, so you can have a quick
and easy meal ready when you need it.

In conclusion, following the Galveston Diet
requires a good understanding of essential
kitchen tools and techniques for preparing
meals. This chapter has provided an
overview of the tools and techniques you
will need to effectively follow the Galveston
Diet, as well as step-by-step instructions for
cooking and preparing meals. Additionally,

it also highlighted how to make the most of leftovers. It is

important to invest in good quality kitchen tools that will make meal preparation easier and more efficient. It's also important to familiarize yourself with different cooking techniques, as they will allow you to prepare a variety of delicious and healthy meals on the Galveston Diet.

When it comes to leftovers, it's important to have a plan for using them before they go bad. This can be done by repurposing them into new dishes or freezing them for later use. This not only saves time and money, but it also helps to reduce food waste.

Overall, by following the Galveston Diet and utilizing essential kitchen tools and techniques, you will be able to prepare delicious and healthy meals that support your weight loss and overall health goals. It may take some time to adjust your cooking skills and recipe to the diet, but once you get the hang of it, it will be a breeze to follow and you will see the benefit in your health.

Recipes range from breakfast bowls to dinner entrees and snacks. Each recipe includes a full list of ingredients, step-by-step instructions, and nutrition information.

Breakfast Bowls

Banana-Coconut Overnight Oats: Start your day off right with this delicious and nutritious breakfast bowl. Combine 1/2 cup rolled oats, 1/2 cup coconut milk, 1/4 teaspoon ground cinnamon, and a pinch of salt in a bowl. Stir in 1 mashed banana and let the mixture sit overnight in the refrigerator. In the morning, top with fresh fruit, shredded coconut, and a drizzle of honey for a sweet start to your day.

Nutrition Information: Calories: 300; Fat: 8g; Carbohydrates: 50g; Protein: 6g; Fiber: 6g

Avocado Toast Bowl: This simple breakfast bowl is packed with flavor and nutrition. Toast 2 slices of whole grain bread until golden brown. Spread each slice with 1/4 mashed avocado and top with a sprinkle of sea salt and freshly ground black pepper. Place the toast on top of a bed of baby spinach leaves and top with 2 tablespoons crumbled feta cheese, 2 tablespoons diced tomatoes, and 2 tablespoons chopped red onion. Drizzle with olive oil for an extra boost of flavor.

Nutrition Information: Calories: 350; Fat: 18g; Carbohydrates: 37g; Protein: 11g; Fiber: 9g

Lunch Entrees

Mediterranean Quinoa Salad Bowls: This light yet filling lunch bowl is full of flavor and nutrition!

Cook 1 cup quinoa according to package instructions then let cool completely before assembling the salad bowls. Divide the quinoa among 4 bowls then top each bowl with 1/4 cup diced cucumber, 1/4 cup diced tomatoes, 2 tablespoons crumbled feta cheese, 2 tablespoons chopped kalamata olives, 2 tablespoons chopped red onion, and 2 tablespoons chopped fresh parsley or basil leaves. Drizzle each bowl with olive oil and freshly squeezed lemon juice then season to taste with sea salt and freshly ground black pepper before serving.

Nutrition Information (per serving): Calories: 250; Fat: 10g; Carbohydrates: 32g; Protein 7g; Fiber 5g

Southwest Chicken Burrito Bowls: These burrito bowls are sure to satisfy your cravings for Mexican food! Heat a large skillet over medium-high heat then add 1 tablespoon of olive oil followed by 1 pound of diced chicken breast or thighs (or both). Cook until chicken is cooked through then season to taste with chili powder, cumin, garlic powder, oregano, sea salt, and freshly ground black pepper before removing from heat to cool slightly before assembling the burrito bowls. Divide cooked chicken among 4 bowls then top each bowl with cooked brown rice or quinoa (or both), black beans (drained & rinsed), shredded lettuce or cabbage mix (or both), diced tomatoes or salsa (or both), guacamole or sliced avocado (or both), shredded cheese (optional), sour cream (optional), jalapeno slices (optional), cilantro leaves (optional). Serve warm or cold depending on preference! Serves 4-6 depending on portion size desired per person.

Nutrition Information (per serving):

Calories 400-500 depending on toppings used;

Fat 15-20 g depending on toppings used;

Carbohydrates 40-50 g depending on toppings used; Protein 25-30 g depending on toppings used ;

Fibre 5-10 g depending on toppings used

CHAPTER FIVE

Dinner Entrees

Baked Salmon & Asparagus Foil Packets: These foil packets are an easy way to get dinner on the table quickly! Preheat oven to 375 degrees F then lines a baking sheet with aluminum foil for easy clean up later! Place 4 salmon fillets onto a prepared baking sheet then season generously with sea salt & freshly ground black pepper before topping each fillet evenly with lemon slices & fresh herbs such as rosemary & thyme if desired. Top each fillet evenly with 12 asparagus spears that have been trimmed & lightly drizzled in olive oil & seasoned lightly if desired. Fold up sides of aluminum foil around the salmon & asparagus so that everything is sealed inside. Bake in preheated oven for 20 minutes or until salmon is cooked through. Serve warm!

Nutrition Information : Calories : 350 ; Fat : 16 g ; Carbohydrates : 8 g ; Protein : 38 g ; Fiber : 3 g

Grilled Vegetable Skewers With Quinoa Pilaf: Fire up the grill for these delicious vegetable skewers! Preheat the grill over medium heat while you prepare your vegetables. Cut bell peppers, zucchini, mushrooms, onions, cherry tomatoes, eggplant, squash, etc into cubes & thread them onto metal skewers. Lightly brush vegetables all over in olive oil & season generously if desired. Grill skewers over medium heat for 10 minutes flipping once halfway through cooking time until vegetables are tender but not mushy. Meanwhile, cook quinoa according to package instructions while the vegetables are grilling. Serve grilled vegetable skewers over cooked quinoa pilaf! Serves 4 - 6 depending on portion size desired per person.

Nutrition Information: Calories: 250 - 300 depending on portion size ;

Fat: 7 - 10 g depending on portion size ;

Carbohydrates: 35 - 45 g depending on portion size; Protein: 8 - 12 g depending on portion size ;

Fibre: 5 - 7 g depending on portion size

Snacks

Roasted Chickpeas With Herbs De Provence: These roasted chickpeas make an excellent snack that's full of protein! Preheat oven to 375 degrees F while you prepare your chickpeas. Drain & rinse one 15-ounce can of chickpeas before patting them dry using paper towels so that they're not too wet when roasting them later. Spread chickpeas out onto a parchment-lined baking sheet & lightly drizzle all over in olive oil before sprinkling generously all over in herbs de Provence seasoning blend if desired along with sea salt & freshly ground black pepper if desired as well before tossing everything together using hands so that everything is evenly coated in seasoning blend before roasting in preheated oven for 20 minutes flipping once halfway through cooking time until golden brown & crispy! Let cool completely before serving! Makes about 3 cups of roasted chickpeas which can be stored in an airtight container at room temperature for up to one week! Enjoy!

Nutrition Information per Serving Size Of ½ Cup Roasted Chickpeas :

Calories 120 ; Fat 3 Grams ;

Carbohydrates 17 Grams ; Protein 5 Grams ;

Fiber 5 Grams

Trail Mix Energy Bites With Dark Chocolate Chips And Coconut Flakes:

These energy bites make an excellent snack that's full of healthy fats from nuts, seeds, dark chocolate chips, coconut flakes, etc! In food processor combine ½ cup almonds , ½ cup cashews , ¼ cup pumpkin seeds , ¼ cup sunflower seeds along with ¼ teaspoon sea salt if desired along with ¼ teaspoon cinnamon if desired as well pulsing several times until ingredients are finely chopped but not too fine like flour consistency should be more like coarsely chopped nuts instead which will help hold energy bites together better when forming them later into balls shape after adding remaining ingredients which will be done next step by adding ½ cup pitted dates along with ¼ cup dark chocolate chips along with ¼ cup unsweetened coconut flakes pulsing several times again until ingredients come together forming dough like consistency which should hold together when pressed between fingers now it's time to form energy bites into balls shape using hands rolling dough between palms into balls shape about one inch diameter placing formed energy bites onto parchment lined baking sheet once finished rolling all energy bites refrigerate at least one hour prior to enjoying them so they can firm up even more making them easier to eat without falling apart enjoy ! Makes about 18 energy bites which can be stored airtight container refrigerator for up two weeks enjoy!

Nutrition Information Per Serving Size Of One Energy Bite Ball About One Inch **Diameter Size Per Ball Approximately : **Calories 80 ; Fat 4 Grams ;

Carbohydrates 9 Grams ; Protein 2 Grams ; Fiber 2 Grams

CHAPTER SIX

Galveston Diet Success Stories

Here are three success stories from individuals who have followed the Galveston Diet and achieved their weight-loss goals:

Sarah, a 32-year-old mother of two, had struggled with her weight for most of her adult life. Despite trying various diets and exercise programs, she could never seem to lose the weight and keep it off. She heard about the Galveston Diet from a friend and decided to give it a try. After following the diet for several months, Sarah was able to lose 25 pounds and improve her overall health. Her motivation for following the diet was to set a good example for her children and to be able to keep up with them as they grew older. Her advice for others following the diet is to stick with it and not to get discouraged if the weight doesn't come off as quickly as you would like.

John, a 42-year-old businessman, had always been active and in good shape, but as he got older, he found it harder to maintain his weight. He was introduced to the Galveston Diet by his doctor and decided to give it a try. After following the diet for several months, John was able to lose 20 pounds and improve his overall health. His motivation for following the diet was to improve his overall health and to be able to keep up with his busy schedule. His advice for others following the diet is to be consistent and not give up if they hit a plateau.

Rachel, a 27-year-old student, had always been overweight and had tried several different diets with little success. She heard about the Galveston Diet from a friend and decided to give it a try. After following the diet for several months, Rachel was able to lose 30 pounds and improve her overall health. Her motivation for following the diet was to improve her self-confidence and to feel better about herself. Her advice for others following the diet is to be patient and not get discouraged if the weight doesn't come off as quickly as you would like.

These stories demonstrate that the Galveston Diet can be effective for weight loss and improving overall health. However, it is important to note that individual results may vary and it is always recommended to consult with a healthcare professional before starting any new diet or exercise program.

conclusion the key points of the Galveston Diet and provides recommendations for how to maintain a healthy lifestyle while following the diet.

The Galveston Diet is a weight loss plan that emphasizes the consumption of high-protein, low-carbohydrate foods.

The key points of the Galveston Diet include:

Reducing carbohydrate intake: The diet focuses on reducing the consumption of carbohydrates, particularly processed and refined carbohydrates, to promote weight loss and improve blood sugar control.

Increasing Protein Intake: The diet encourages the consumption of high-quality protein sources, such as meat, fish, eggs, and dairy, to help individuals feel full and satisfied while also promoting muscle growth and repair.

Limiting Processed Foods: The Galveston Diet discourages the consumption of processed foods, as they are often high in added sugars and preservatives that can be detrimental to health.

Incorporating Healthy Fats: The diet promotes the consumption of healthy fats, such as olive oil, avocado, and nuts, to help individuals feel full and satisfied while also providing important nutrients for overall health.

Prioritizing Whole Foods: The Galveston Diet encourages the consumption of whole, unprocessed foods, such as fruits, vegetables, and whole grains, as they are often more nutrient-dense than their processed counterparts.

To maintain a healthy lifestyle while following the Galveston Diet, it is important to:

Before making any significant dietary changes, speak with a medical practitioner.

Ensure that you are getting enough fruits, vegetables, and whole grains, despite the low-carb focus of the diet

Make sure you are getting enough fiber, as it is an important nutrient for gut health.

Balance your protein intake, as consuming too much protein can be harmful to the kidneys

Consider taking a multivitamin supplement to ensure that you are getting enough vitamins and minerals.

Additional support and advice can be found through a registered dietitian, who can help you create a personalized meal plan that meets your individual needs and goals. Websites such as the American Dietetic Association (ADA) and the Academy of Nutrition and Dietetics (AND) can also provide reliable information on healthy eating and weight loss.

It's important to note that the Galveston Diet is not well-studied and there's no scientific evidence to support its claims. Before making any significant dietary changes, it's crucial to speak with a trained dietician or a healthcare provider.

Printed in Great Britain
by Amazon

21135584R00045